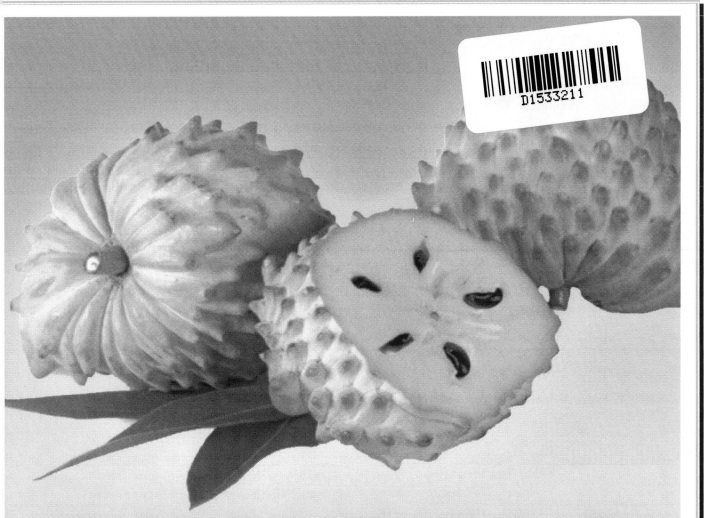

GRAVIOLA
and
How It Can Health the Cancer

GRAVIOLA
And how it can
heal the cancer

By GyoBy

Preface

Cancer is second only to cardiovascular disease as the leading cause of death in the Western world. Although Cancer is primarily a disease of the elderly with more than 60% of deaths from cancer occurring in those over the age of 65, cancer can strike even the youngest of children.

Cancer appears to occur when the growth of cells in the body is out of control and cells divide too rapidly. Cancer can develop in almost any organ or tissue, such as the lung, colon, breast, skin, bones, or nerve tissue.

"The time has come" - how many times we are hearing this sentence, nevertheless it is true because we are living in times of huge challenges, changes and shifts where secrets of many different aspect of life are getting revealed to be known by the public - people also are more courageous to speak out what all should know and YES, if millions KNOW a fact, those who are hiding solutions, will have to surrender.

TABLE OF CONTENTS

INTRODUCTION

Graviola also known as Annona muricata, soursop or guananbaba, the possible Graviola cancer cure has been under investigation since the 1940s. This tropical plant grows in Central and South America and has been purposely grown for its healing properties for more than three centuries. The bark, fruit, leaves and roots have been utilized in folk medicines mainly as a sedative. However, native South American healers have used the plant to improve ailments such as heart complaints, arthritis, liver problems, fevers and asthma.

The National Cancer Institute carried out the first modern clinical research on Graviola in 1976. Tests done at Perdue University found that prostate, lung and pancreatic cancerous cells were killed by the leaves of the Graviola plant. Further studies were conducted to investigate the chemical effects of the plant in laboratory tests, however tests on humans or animals are required to create conclusive results. Studies in Korea resulted in findings that cells from colon cancer where destroyed more effectively 10,000 times stronger - using Graviola than Adriamycin, a popular chemotherapy drug. Taken in isolation and with the □uest continuing to find a cure for cancer Graviola certainly seems to be very effective.

There are known side effects from chemotherapy which is used on tumors like mesothelioma cancer, such as hair loss and nausea. However, Graviola only targeted and killed the carcinogenic cells leaving normal healthy cells alone, much more preferable than toxic drugs which can kill the cancer but also the healthy cells. Cancers such as malignant mesothelioma and peritoneal mesothelioma are aggressive cancers caused by exposure to asbestos, a naturally occurring mineral used in building. Its use has now been banned.

In traditional native folk medicine, the seeds of Graviola are utilized in the removal of parasites in the human body. Jamaicans and West Indians eat the fruit to stop diarrhea and lower fevered body temperatures. Brazilians make a tea from Graviola to relieve liver complaints and extract oils from the seeds to improve rheumatic conditions and arthritis. In Guyana the leaves are made into a tea and drank for a healthy heart and as a sedative.

The Graviola herb has shown promising results and the active ingredients are called Annonaceous acetogenins. In test tubes they have aggressive anticancer results and only a small amount is needed to produce positive effects 1 part in 100,000,000 for example.

The Graviola tree cancer cure is still under trial but, worldwide, there are more than two thousand varieties of plants in the Annonaceae family and the potential for further cures to serious diseases is clearly exciting. Graviola supplements and Graviola extract are available to aid well-being and taken as a general healthful tonic for the body. The fruit is high in carbohydrates especially fructose and contains significant vitamins C, B1 and B2. So, it seems that there is hope, however, more in depth research needs to be conducted to produce a definitive graviola cancer cure.

According to Cancer Tutor, the use of graviola with alternative natural cancer cure, Protocel, can increase the effectiveness of Protocel but it is a risky treatment that is not recommended at all for brain cancer patients. Graviola attacks cancer cells by cutting off their energy supply. The problem is that graviola extracts are easily available over the counter and most cancer patients are taking self prescribed medicines. It is extremely important to consult a doctor and take medication as recommended by them. A lot of oncologists are gravitating towards combining cancer therapy with natural remedies for cancer to prevent cancer from resurfacing. However, for stage III and stage IV patients, chemotherapy is the only option for increasing their life span.

Apart from inflicting symptoms similar to Alzheimer's, graviola can also result in the destruction of digestive and intestinal lining, especially in people who do not have any parasitic ailments. Most manufacturers provide a list of symptoms that may occur post graviola intake but caution must be advised. It is important not to trust sources on the internet blindly, unless supported by a recognized cancer research institute.

PLANT CHEMICALS

Many active compounds and chemicals have been found in graviola, as scientists have been studying its properties since the 1940s. Most of the research on graviola focuses on a novel set of chemicals called Annonaceous acetogenins. Graviola produces these natural compounds in its leaf and stem, bark, and fruit seeds. Three separate research groups have confirmed that these chemicals have significant antitumorous properties and selective toxicity against various types of cancer cells (without harming healthy cells) publishing eight clinical studies on their findings. Many of the acetogenins have demonstrated selective toxicity to tumor cells at very low dosages as little as 1 part per million. Four studies were published in 1998 which further specify the chemicals and acetogenins in graviola which are demonstrating the strongest anticancerous, antitumorous, and antiviral properties. In a 1997 clinical study, novel alkaloids found in graviola fruit exhibited antidepressive effects in animals.

Annonaceous acetogenins are only found in the Annonaceae family (to which graviola belongs). These chemicals in general have been documented with antitumorous, antiparasitic, insecticidal, and antimicrobial activities. Mode of action studies in three separate laboratories have recently determined that these acetogenins are superb inhibitors of enzyme processes that are only found in the membranes of cancerous tumor cells. This is why they are toxic to cancer cells but have no toxicity to healthy cells. Purdue University, in West Lafayette, Indiana, has conducted a great deal of the research on the acetogenins, much of which, has been funded by The National Cancer Institute and/or the National Institute of Health (NIH). Thus far, Purdue University and/or its staff have filed at least nine U.S. and/or international patents on their work around the antitumorous and insecticidal properties and uses of these acetogenins.

In 1997, Purdue University published information with promising news that several of the Annonaceous acetogenins were not only are effective in killing tumors that have proven resistant to anti-cancer agents, but also seem to have a special affinity for such resistant cells." In several interviews after this information was publicized, the head pharmacologist in Purdue's research explained how this worked. As he explains it, cancer cells that survive chemotherapy can develop resistance to the agent originally used as well as to other, even unrelated, drugs. This phenomenon is called multi-drug resistance (MDR). One of the main ways that cancer cells develop resistance to chemotherapy drugs is by creating an intercellular pump which is capable of pushing anticancer agents out of the cell before they can kill it. On average, only about two percent of the cancer cells in any given person might develop this pump but they are the two percent that can eventually grow and expand to create multi-drug-resistant tumors. Some of the latest research on acetogenins reported that they were capable of shutting down these intercellular pumps, thereby killing multi-drug-resistant tumors. Purdue researchers reported that the acetogenins preferentially killed multi-drug-resistant cancer cells by blocking the transfer of ATP the chief source of cellular energy into them. A tumor cell needs energy to grow and reproduce, and a great deal more to run its pump and expel attacking agents. By inhibiting energy to the cell , it can no longer run its pump. When acetogenins block ATP to the tumor cell over time, the cell no longer has enough energy to operate sustaining processes and it dies. Normal cells seldom develop such a pump; therefore, they don't require large amounts of energy to run a pump and, generally, are not adversely affected by ATP inhibitors. Purdue researchers reported that 14 different acetogenins tested thus far demonstrate potent ATP-blocking properties (including several found only in graviola). They also reported that 13 of these 14 acetogenins tested were more potent against MDR breast cancer cells than all three of the standard drugs (adriamycin, vincristine, and vinblastine) they used as controls.

The Annonaceous acetogenins discovered in graviola thus far include: annocatalin, annohexocin, annomonicin, annomontacin, annomuricatin A & B, annomuricin A thru E, annomutacin, annonacin, annonacinone, annopentocin A thru C, cis-annonacin, cis-corossolone, cohibin A thru D, corepoxylone, coronin, corossolin, corossolone, donhexocin, epomuricenin A & B, gigantetrocin, gigantetrocin A & B, gigantetrocinone, gigantetronenin, goniothalamicin, iso-annonacin, javoricin, montanacin, montecristin, muracin A thru G, muricapentocin, muricatalicin, muricatalin, muri-catenol, muricatetrocin A & B muricatin D, muricatocin A thru C muricin H, muricin I, muricoreacin, murihexocin 3, murihexocin A thru C, murihexol, murisolin, robustocin, rolliniastatin 1 & 2, saba-delin, solamin, uvariamicin I & IV, xylomaticin

BIOLOGICAL ACTIVITES AND CLINICAL RESEARCH

In an 1976 plant screening program by the National Cancer Institute, graviola leaves and stem showed active toxicity against cancer cells and researchers have been following up on these findings since. Thus far, specific acetogenins in graviola and/or extracts of graviola have been reported to be selectively toxic in vitro to these types of tumor cells: lung carcinoma cell lines; human breast solid tumor lines; prostate adenocarcinoma; pancreatic carcinoma cell lines; colon adenocarcinoma cell lines; liver cancer cell lines; human lymphoma cell lines; and multi-drug resistant human breast adenocarcinoma. Researchers in Taiwan reported in 2003 that the main graviola acetogenin, annonacin, was highly toxic to ovarian, cervical, breast, bladder and skin cancer cell lines at very low dosages saying; " annonacin is a promising anti-cancer agent and worthy of further animal studies and, we would hope, clinical trials."

An interesting in vivo study was published in March of 2002 by researchers in Japan, who were studying various acetogenins found in several species of plants. They inoculated mice with lung cancer cells. One third received nothing (the control group), one third received the chemotherapy drug adriamycin, and one third received the main graviola acetogenin, annonacin (at a dosage of 10 mg/kg). At the end of two weeks, five of the six in the untreated control group were still alive and lung tumor sizes were then measured. The adriamycin group showed a 54.6% reduction of tumor mass over the control group but 50% of the animals had died from toxicity (three of six). The mice receiving annonacin were all still alive, and the tumors were inhibited by 57.9%

slightly better than adriamycin and without toxicity. This led the researchers to summarize; "This suggested that annonacin was less toxic in mice. On considering the antitumor activity and toxicity, annonacin might be used as a lead to develop a potential anticancer agent."

CURRENT PRACTICAL USES

Cancer research is ongoing on these important Annona plants and plant chemicals, as several pharmaceutical companies and universities continue to research, test, patent, and attempt to synthesize these chemicals into new chemotherapeutic drugs. In fact, graviola seems to be following the same path as another well known cancer drug – Taxol. From the time researchers first discovered an antitumorous effect in the bark of the pacific yew tree and a novel chemical called taxol was discovered in its bark it took thirty years of research by numerous pharmaceutical companies, universities, and government agencies before the first FDA-approved Taxol drug was sold to a cancer patient (which was based on the natural taxol chemical they found in the tree bark).

With graviola, it has taken researchers almost 10 years to successfully synthesize (chemically reproduce) the main antitumorous chemical, annonacin. These acetogenin chemicals have a unique waxy center and other unique molecular energy properties which thwarted earlier attempts, and at least one major pharmaceutical company gave up in the process (despite knowing how active the natural chemical was against tumors). Now that scientists have the ability to recreate this chemical and several other active acetogenins in the laboratory, the next step is to change the chemical just enough (without losing any of the antitumorous actions in the process) to become a novel chemical which can be patented and turned into a new patented cancer drug. (Naturally-occurring plant chemicals cannot be patented.) Thus far, scientists seem to be thwarted again every time they change the chemical enough to be patentable, they lose much of the antitumorous actions. Like the development of taxol, it may well take government agenies like the National Cancer Institute and the National Institute of Health to step forward and launch full-scale human cancer research on the synthesized unpatentable natural plant chemical (which will allow any pharmaceutical company to develop a cancer drug utilizing the research as happened with taxol) to be able to make this promising therapy available to cancer patients in a timely fashion.

In the meantime, many cancer patients and health practitioners are not waiting… they are adding the natural leaf and stem of graviola (with over 40 documented naturally-occurring acetogenins including annonacin) as a complementary therapy to their cancer protocols. After all, graviola has a long history of safe use as a herbal remedy for other conditions for many years, and research indicates that the antitumorous acetogenins are selectively toxic to just cancer cells and not healthy cells and in miniscule amounts. While research confirms that these antitumorous acetogenins also occur in high amounts in the fruit seeds and roots of graviola, different alkaloid chemicals in the seeds and roots have shown some preliminary in vitro neurotoxic effects. Researchers have suggested that these alkaloids might be linked to atypical Parkinson's disease in countries where the seeds are employed as a common herbal parasite remedy. Therefore, using the seeds and root of graviola is not recommended at this time.

The therapuetic dosage of graviola leaf, (which offers just as high of an amount of acetogenins as the root and almost as much as the seed) is reported to be 2-3 grams taken 3 or 4 times daily.

Graviola products (capsules and tinctures) are becoming more widely available in the U.S. market, and now offered under several different manufacturer's labels in health food stores. As one of graviola's mechanisms of action is to deplete ATP energy to cancer cells, combining it with other supplements and natural products which increase or enhance cellular ATP may reduce the effect of graviola. The main supplement which increases ATP is a common antioxidant called Coenzyme Q10 and for this reason, it should be avoided when taking graviola.

Graviola is certainly a promising natural remedy and one that again emphasizes the importance of preserving our remaining rainforest ecosystems. Perhaps if enough people believe that the possible cure for cancer truly is locked away in a rainforest plant we will take the steps needed to protect our remaining rainforests from destruction. One researcher studying graviola summarized this idea eloquently: "At the time of preparation of this current review, over 350 Annonaceous acetogenins have been isolated from 37 species. Our preliminary efforts show that about 50%, of over 80 Annonaceous species screened, are significantly bioactive and are worthy of fractionation; thus, this class of compounds can be expected to continue to grow at an exponential rate in the future, provided that financial support for such research efforts can be found. With the demise of the world's tropical rain forests, such work is compelling before the great chemical diversity, contained within these endangered species, is lost."

SCIENTIFIC RESULTS ON GRAVIOLA

The Graviola Fruit is already under research since the late 39 of last century - At that Time the science found out that the plant has components, natural principles and properties called "Annonacaeous Acetogenins", natural chemicals that are confirmed to be highly effective against many kind of tumor cells with components that are found as toxins that kills the cancer cells in a very specific way. Simply spoken Graviola has components that are able to isolate every cancer cell, to build a kind of bubble around it avoiding that the cancer cell can get any further nutrient, so it dies. The dead cancer cells are eliminated by the own body system without any side effects. Those components are hidden in all parts of the tree and in different combination they are used for many different kind of disease. They are documented as anti-microbus, anti-parasitic, antitumorous, anti-cancerous, anti-depressive and anti-spasmodic. Several study results have been published but few people reacted.

Since 1976 profound researches of the National Cancer Institute of the USA resulted in curing an "Adenocarcinoma" of the large intestine after short time. The therapeutic effect confirmed the power of Graviola and her components. This powerful component has been discovered by the German Research Scientist and Oncologist Helmut Keller and with three more Scientists they realized many studies on Graviola. As the Plant does NOT ALLOW any chemical process without losing the healing powers never nobody got to know about this effective cancer treatment. WHY??? - because it only works in natural form and a plant cannot be patented in any form, so the Pharmaceutical World and the Monopoles could not get any profit from it and that is the reason they hided the information.

Result:

Graviola contains very active, cytotoxic effects against cancer cells with a chemo therapeutic power that is 10.000 x stronger as Adriamicin, the drug that is used for traditional Chemo Therapy, without any kind of side effects!

(Since a while the HSI is offering now the copies of the results that can be bought for 25,00USD)

After the confirmation that Graviola can cure naturally Cancer the National Health Institute has indicated 20 Labs to studies the plant during 20 years without any result to transform the active principles into a valid remedy. At the end they gave up and let the miraculous findings in the drawer of their institutes.

Since 1996 other groups of scientists did researches on Graviola and found out that the fruit possesses characteristics against tumor formation and that it produces selective toxins against different kinds of cancer cells, without attacking healthy cells. They confirmed the findings of their results were published 8 different clinical studies.

The different studies of different laboratories resulted in incredible findings that the Acetogenines of Graviola have an unbeatable component in prevention of enzyme formations, which are only found in the diaphragm by tumors and cancer cells. That is the reason, why they are poisonous only for cancer cells without attacking healthy cells. The Acetonines recognize the sick cells isolates the individual cancer cells and for missing nutrients the cancer cell dies.

In the year 1997 a small group of scientists found out, that Graviola contains also alkaloids which have an anti-depressive effect. In the same year the PARDU UNIVERSITY published the information that they discovered even more powers within Graviola. Their clinical studies confirmed that the "Annonacae Acetonine" in Graviola are so effective, that they do not only kill normal cancer cells, but that they are also very effective in killing those cancer cells that are resistant on Chemo Therapy. This investigation explained how that is possible: Those cancer cells that survive the Chemo Therapy are developing resistance against many other kind of drugs, called Multi-Drug-Resistant (MDR) what makes them immune against any treatment and leads the patient 100% to death.

After 20 Year of research the Pharma Industry got aware of the Plant and started research by their own seeking a form and way to transform the active principles and components into a cancer remedy. They also failed. Graviola does not allow any kind of chemical reproduction. It is reconfirmed that Graviola only works as it grows in nature and it beats cancer better then any synthetic drug or heavy poison rays. Until today many different groups of scientists are still researching to create a similar product as Annonacins and it still works only like it grown in Nature.

All that information has been kept in secret because Pharmacies could not transform it into something that would give them a huge profit. So they gave proof that they are not really interested in heal people but in making huge profits from those who are already sufficiently hidden by the disease itself. Why would somebody create so many unnecessary pain when there is something much stronger and without any life threatening side effect.

At the end of the nineties one of the Scientists who was part of one of the research teams broke the silence for reasons of consciousness and some of the reports were accessible for the medicine world. Simultaneously some people from Brazil got kind of divine guidance to go to the Amazon and to study the Plants of the Rainforest. They were integrating the native people to learn from them as their knowledge about healing plants of the Rainforest is reaching back in time for many centuries.

The good thing is that for one time in this world the science is NOT finding a way of manipulation - the power of healing cancer lies in Graviola and several further plants that God preserved to be used like the Almighty lets it grow. It is a blessing for Mankind and a gift from Mother Earth - A wake up call to become conscious and to start honoring the gifts we have forgotten that they exist. When we destroy the rainforests we destroy the lungs of our planet and without oxygen all life will die. We need to open up our hearts to understand that all what we experience has a solution and all what we suffer of different kind of disease has a natural way of cure in nature.

A FRIENDLY SKEPTIC LOOKS AT GRAVIOLA

Hardly a day goes by that I am not asked for my opinion of some new cancer treatment. When it comes to evaluating the merits of any treatment, conventional or unconventional, I try to maintain a mindset of "friendly skepticism." On the one hand, I remain receptive to all promising new approaches. Lord knows, conventional oncology leaves much to be desired and society desperately needs new ideas. On the other hand, we live in a world filled with hustlers and opportunists, and we have to be constantly on our guard against expensive and dangerous rip-offs. We want to protect patients while at the same time not discouraging innovative researchers.

A reader once called me a "soft-core □uackbuster". Although he later retracted the charge, I have to confess that I wasn't terribly upset at the label. As I see it, quackery exists on both sides of the medical divide: neither conventional medicine nor alternative medicine is immune from this scourge or has a monopoly on probity. A major problem with the self-proclaimed "□uackbusters" is that their one-sided and tendentious attacks on alternative medicine leave the impression that conventional medicine is the only valid way of treating most forms of cancer. They come across as knee-jerk defenders of a status quo that genuinely needs to be reformed, not supported unquestioningly. On the other hand, I am wary of exaggerated claims made for any cancer treatments, whether those treatments originate in orthodox or alternative medicine, because such overblown claims are often based on (let us be generous) commercial considerations rather than solid science.

A case in point is an herbal treatment called Graviola. This burst onto the Internet in early 1999 and is now incorporated into many patients' regimens. An increasing number of alternative practitioners are recommending it to their patients.

What exactly is Graviola? It is a common name for Annona muricata, also known as soursop or Brazilian paw-paw. This is a small, upright evergreen tree growing 15 to 18 feet in height with large, glossy dark green leaves. (It is not to be confused with Asimina triloba, a deciduous tree of the eastern and southeast United States .)

Graviola is indigenous to warm tropical areas in the Americas , including the Amazon. It produces a 6-to-9 inch, heart-shaped edible fruit, yellow-green in color, with white flesh. This is sold in tropical markets under the name guanabana or Brazilian cherimoya. It is said to be is excellent for making drinks and sherbets and, though slightly sour-acid, can be eaten out-of-hand.

If you enter the term "Graviola" into Google you come up with an amazing 12,300 citations, over 2,000 of which relate to cancer. You also get a rash of sidebar advertisements such as "A great product to fight cancer," "Graviola helps to fight cancer," and "How Millions Beat Cancer," presumably with the help of this herb. It is reputedly "10,000 times stronger in killing colon cancer than Adriamycin, a commonly used chemotherapeutic drug" and has the ability to "hunt down and destroy prostate, lung, breast, colon, and pancreatic cancers... leaving healthy cells alone!"

These are formidable claims. Adriamycin (doxorubicin) is one of the most powerful (and toxic) drugs in chemotherapy. Adriamycin was discovered in Italy in the 1970s, hence the "Adria-tic" name. I well remember its introduction into oncology and how it revolutionized the treatment of several forms of cancer. But now, we are told, an herb has come to light that is not only as powerful as Adriamycin, but 10,000 times more powerful, and non-toxic to boot. The mind reels. Reading this statement, one cannot wait to find out more about this herbal product and how it could be used to help cancer patients. One pictures the evil demon Cancer, beaten and cringing in its corner, knowing that its days on earth are numbered.

I don't know who first penned these effusive statements about Graviola but the claims have taken on a life of their own. I found two dozen other websites that contained the exact phrasing about Graviola being "10,000 times stronger than Adriamycin," all equally unsupported by scientific references. It seems that astounding claims concerning cancer cures spread like a virus from Website to Website.

The phrase "annonaceous acetogenins" gave a new and promising starting point. Indeed, this term yielded 121 citations in PubMed. A lot of these were about the chemical constituents of the fruit. But taken cumulatively, one gathers that there is indeed a class of very interesting and potentially useful compounds in various branches of the Annona family. To quote scientists at

Purdue University's highly regarded School of Pharmacy, "Annonaceous acetogenins are an extremely potent class of compounds, and their inhibition of cell growth can be selective for cancerous cells and also effective for drug resistant cancer cells, while exhibiting only minimal toxicity to 'normal' non-cancerous cells" (Oberlies 1995). Graviola thus joins the list of hundreds of other biologically active plants that are of potential importance to the future of medicine.

Further searching in PubMed revealed that it was in fact scientists at Purdue who had first come up with the widely-circulated "more powerful than Adriamycin" claim. Here is what Dr. X.X. Liu and colleagues stated in 1999: "Annoglacins A and B were selectively 1000 and 10,000 times, respectively, more potent than Adriamycin against the human breast carcinoma (MCF-7) and pancreatic carcinoma (PACA-2) cell lines in our panel of six human solid tumor cell lines."

This is very exciting in principle. However, to an inquiring, healthily skeptical mind, several questions immediately suggest themselves. One is, how much "annoglacin B" is found in a typical Graviola capsule purchased over the Internet? Quite probably it is infinitessimally small. Also lost in the promotional hoo-hah is the fact that the particular annoglacins investigated by Dr Liu and colleagues were derived not from Graviola at all but from a related, but entirely different, species, Annona glabra. This is a Polynesian tree called the pond or alligator apple.

My understanding of the term "clinical studies" is that they necessarily involve the treatment of human beings (or, more inclusively, pet and farm animals). Webster says that the term 'clinical' is an observation that "involves or is based on direct observation of the patient." The Cancerweb dictionary states that the word 'clinical' pertains to or is founded on "actual observation and treatment of patients, as distinguished from theoretical or basic sciences."

Sadly, Graviola has now entered the netherworld of alternative cancer treatments. It promises much based on real, but very preliminary, scientific facts. Now its reputation has been tarnished by misstatements and over-promotion. Is there any way for a promising treatment to find its way back from the Purgatory of Cancer Cure-Alls? Or shall we remain forever in the dark about the merits of such treatments? Thousands of cancer patients are waiting for an answer to that riddle.

USES OF GRAVIOLA

Botanical Description

Graviola is a small, upright tropical evergreen tree, 5-6 m high, with large, glossy, dark green leaves. It produces a large, heart-shaped, edible fruit that is 15-23 cm in diameter, is yellow-green in color and has white flesh inside. The fruit is popular in South America.

Ethnobotanical Uses

All parts of the graviola tree have been used medicinally in traditional herbal medicine. Traditional herbal medicine practitioners have attributed graviola with the following properties and actions: anthelmintic, antiparasitic, antipyretic, sedative, antispasmodic, nervine, hypotensive, anticonvulsant and digestive.

Indian Tribes use Graviola as medicine since Centuries

Graviola counts with a very long history in the tribal herbal natural medicine. There are Healing substances in every part of the plant: a part of the powerful effects of the fruit we find high effective substances in the leaves, the roots, the trunk, the bark and the seeds. Indian Tribes know about the value of that miraculous tree and they are using the different parts tor multiple and diverse diseases and health Imbalances. Some examples:

- *Flower:* Bronchitis, cough.
- *Fruit:* Colitis, diarrhea, dysentery, fevers, hydropsy, juice, lactogogue, mouth sores, parasites, tranquilizer.
- *Seeds:* Astringent, carminative, emetic, head lice, insecticide, parasites, skin parasites, worms.
- *Bark:* Asthenia, asthma, childbirth, cough, diabetesgrippe, heart tonic, hypertension, nervine, parasites, sedative, spasms.
- *Leaf:* Abscesses, arthritis pain, asthenia, asthma, astringent, bronchitis, catarrh, colic, cough, diabetes, diuretic, dysentery, edema, fever, gallbladder disorders, grippe, heart, hypertension, indigestion, infections, intestinal worms, lactogogue, liver disorders, malaria, nervine, nervousness, neuralgia, palpitations, parasites, parturition, rashes, rheumatism, ringworm, sedative, skin disorders, spasms, styptic, tonic, tran□uilizer, tumors, ulcers, worms.
- *Root:* Diabetes, sedative, spasms
- *Rootbark:* Calmative, diabetes, spasms

In Brazil Roots, Trunk and leaves are used as sedative tee and against nervousness, in other Latin America countries as sedative and as heart tonic medium, also for Diabetes. The leave tee is also used for lever problems and mixed with olive oil it is used for Rheumatism, Arthritis and

Osteoarthritis pain in Peru. In Brazil they prepare a mixture out of an immature fruit mixed with Olive oil as extern treatment against Arthritis and Rheumatism.

Leaves are also used against Parasites in Brazil and against Catarrh in Peru.

Fruit, Seeds and Leaves are applied against fever, all kind of parasites, worms, diarrhea, in Brazil also to help increasing the milk of women after giving birth.

In other countries such as Haiti, West Indies and Jamaica are using Graviola as anti spasmodic, sedative, coughs and flu, as nerve strengthening tee, for asthma, hypertension and all kind of parasites, diarrhea and problems at childbirth.

Latin America:

Brazil:

Abscesses, Tumors, Edemas, Worms, all kind of Parasites, Bronchitis, Breathing Difficulties, Coughs, Diabetes, Digestive Imbalances, Dysentery, Intestine Parasites, the Intestinal/Colic Attacks, Fever, Liver Problems, Neuralgias, Nervousness, general Body Pain, Rheumatism, Tetanus

Peru

Tumors of all kind, Intern Ulcers, Parasites, Lice, Hypertension Diabetes, Dysentery, Indigestion, Inflammation, Flu, Liver Disorders, Spasms, Fever and as a Sedative

Panama:

Tumors, Ulcers, Parasites, Worms, Digestive Disorders (Dyspepsia), Diarrhea and Kidney Problems: Renal Insufficiency - Renal Failure

Mexico:

Tapeworm, Indigestion, Diarrhea, Dysentery, Fever, Chest Colds, Ringworm, Scurvy, Styptic (bleeding)

The Caribbean:

Colds, chills, fever, flu, diarrhea, indigestion, nervousness, palpitations, rash, spasms, skin disease, and as a sedative and calmative agent

Curacao:

Gallbladder Problems, Nervousness, as a Sedative and Calmative Agent, Childbirth

Haiti:

Parasites, Lice, Flu, Digestive Sluggishness, Diarrhea, Fever, Coughs, Pain, Weakness, Wounds, Pellagra, Nervousness, Cardiopathy, Spasms, Sedative, Lactation Aid after Childbirth,

Jamaica:

Parasites, Worms, Asthma, Fevers, Heart Disease, Hypertension, Lactation Aid after Childbirth, Nervousness, Sedative, Spasms, Tetanus, Water Retention and general Weakness,

Trinidad:

Ringworms, Blood Cleaning Agent, Hypertension, Palpitations, Fainting, Insomnia, Lactation Aid after Childbirth, Flu,

USA:

Cancer, Tumors, Ulcers, Fungal Infections, Intestine Parasites, Hypertension, Depression

Asia - Malaysia

Furuncles, Coughs, Colds, Diarrhea, Dermatosis, Hypertension, Rheumatism, and to Reduce Bleeding

British West Indies:

Tumors, Intestine Parasites, Asthma, Childbirth, Lactation Aid, Hypertension

Other Countries:

Cancer, Kidney Problems, Bladder Insufficiency, Liver Disorders, Dysentery, Malaria, Stomach Problems, Ringworm, Lice, Parasites, Childbirth, Asthma, Hypertension, Heart Disease, Arthritis, Scurvy and as a Sedative

The traditional use of graviola has been recorded in herbal medicine systems in the following countries:

Amazonia, Barbados, Borneo, Brazil, Cook Islands, Curacao, Dominica, Guatemala, Guam, Guyana, Haiti, Jamaica, Madagascar, Malaysia, Peru, Suriname, Togo and West Indies.

Traditional Preparation: The therapeutic dosage is reported to be 2 g three times daily in capsules or tablets. A standard infusion (one cup 3 times daily) or a 4:1 standard tincture (2–4 ml three times daily) can be substituted if desired.

NUTRITIVE VALUES OF GRAVIOLA

Minerals

Iron, potassium, calcium, copper, magnesium, manganese, sodium, phosphorus, sulfur, Selenium, zinc,

Vitamines

Vitamin A, Vitamin B1, Vitamin B2, Vitamin B3, Vitamin C

In addition

Dietary fibers, Tannin, Proteins, Lipides

Ethno-medical Uses of Graviola in different Tropical Countries and USA

NATIVE WISDOM

After learning about ethnological medicine and their high evolved knowledge we should ask ourselves who is more advanced. They have no hospitals and they have NO CANCER or did you ever see a Native in a Cancer Department of a Hospital? They do not have Laboratories, they don't transform any plant into a pill and they are heal.

The Natives still show us today how to live with nature and how nature provides all what we need for a healthy life. What do we as the so called Civilized World with Nature and with ourselves? We allow destructive exploitation, depletion, exhaustive cultivation, robber economy, not only with Mother Nature but also with our own lives. We burn the candle at two ends disrespecting the holiness of our body. We abuse a maximum and the end is deadly disease. Is that a wonder? No it is just a conse□uence of our issues, our habits, our believe systems and our actions, of out thoughts, words and the ability to look away when things are not in harmony with the cosmic order. We just don't care when it does not hit us personally. To heal really we have to heal ALL THE REALMS we are living in otherwise we only get a momentum cure. Can you feel that? It is NOT a question of understanding but of feeling!!!!! We shot our feelings down

You go against your feelings and you get sick!!!

How many times a day we do that???? We have to come back to the heart and stand up to safe the natural resources that are still intact like the rainforest as biggest source of healing plants that exists in our world.

A German Doctor made holiday in the Amazon Region and he was wondering how many natural remedies are there on the market. He took some of the to try and as I started to teach in Germany about Graviola and the Rainforest he showed up and said: I am director of a Hospital and I was looking for a way to make people the Amazonian Healing Powers available. I our Hospital we have a new system and are open for alternative healing methods. We offer open Seminaries and you can come whenever you want to talk about cancer and other disease. I did for Diabetes..... it was amazing

So the Western Countries are learning about Graviola and the Healing Powers of Graviola, the miraculous fruit that brings never ending surprises to people with cancer and other heavy disease. Graviola is a chance for all those who are hidden by Cancer or one of the other diseases of civilization.

Graviola is not only a miracle against cancer cells, but has also components (results of researches) that can eliminate other chemicals like cortisone, drugs and all kind poisons in our body. This is UNIQUE as Cortisone remains into people's bodies forever with the horrendous side effect that people are gaining weight fro nothing. Graviola is the power of life that is able to clean all poisons we are exposed today in our daily life in air, water and nutrients. It has the amazing natural potency to clean and to regenerate our body cells. Just remember that our body is the Holy Temple of Life that deserves all our respect because the body makes us the gift to be alive and to experience this wonderful personal journey on this beautiful planet, to have fun and grow in all senses when we maintain us in a healthy state.

This Plant and many others are a gift of Divine Source and Mother Earth preserved for our times to remember the love we should have for our divine vehicle, for ourselves and for all life. Divine Source and Mother Earth have the medium for people who have lost faith in the daily battle for survival.

This fruit has the form of a huge heart to show you even by its form that only the heart can heal without any kind of human manipulation, pure and natural like it is given.

A little insight of my own experiences:

As Multi-Dimensional Free Way Healer I learned to go straight to the cause of a disease that is created by denying feelings, psychic shocks, and heavy experiences on heart and soul level as well as body misuse of any kind. It can be karmic origin or even living on a place that is over poisoned by electricity or environmental. Nevertheless we can never get sick when our body defense is working properly and that opens the door to all what we experience. The way of cause and effect never fails and even incurable disease is curable by cosmic law. I always was driven to the Rainforest and I knew deep within that some kind of cure for the physical body should exist in that huge natural pharmacy of Mother Earth. I asked God to get something into my hands that helps people faster to understand and faster to heal so they can learn on big scale and not just one by one.

7 years ago - I was at about to travel to Germany and the day before a friend of my spiritual group from years ago over sudden crossed my way and she asked me when I am going to travel again to Germany and if I could help the next time I go to open an enterprise that sells Amazon Natural Nutrients that are a power house of healing and there is nobody who speaks well German. Well, the word Amazon was hitting me like an electric shock and I was just going the next day... Is this the answer of my prayers I thought. After one week something drove me to get in touch and I felt the obligation to call. The representative came to present the products, 7 at that time. He started to explain each one and as I held the bottle of a mixture of Graviola and 6 other anti cancerous components in my hands instantaneously my entire body was increasing tremendous heat waves and source transmitted: that is what you have asked for. Of course I studied all I had to and stood in Germany for 9 month to get the information out fighting the meanings and beliefs of traditional cancer cure.

There are so many cases I was testimony of that it would fill books and it would made you cry as it does with 100s of people when they hear at the annual gathering people telling their stories of survival in the last moment - their despair facing death and their families without a penny left because no assurance would take the bills anymore - family selling everything they have to safe a beloved one.

One friend of mine Brazilian Plastic Surgery Specialist got Leukemia Myeloid and the needed urgently a cell transplant - she was on a list number 989 - I past 4 month with her working on her and finally we could access the products and the doctor of the enterprise said to her: You know that you are in the hands of God? Yes - but nevertheless we will give it a try - you got to take 5 different products and we found a sponsor - today she has a foundation for abandoned animals - she left her wheel chair behind and she is fine!!!!

All those experiences are divine one by one but I think that more people need to know about it - from mouth to mouth it is just to slow - there are so many people suffering for nothing. The Lady who became director of the German enterprise had 5 types of cancer - 5 children - her best friend a director of a Hospital - he told her to go home and to spend the last time with her children - that his art has come to an end and that he is so sorry. At home a friend passed by and told her about those products - she loves life and she took one product only - after a week she felt stronger - her life powers came back she felt that she could make it and she said she would only go and show up front of her doctor and friend when she was fine. After 6 month she visited him in the hospital he cried and asked what she did - she talked about the products and halleluiah the doctor today is working in his hospital with those products too. There is not only hope THERE IS HEALING OUT THERE and people need to be informed!

As we learned, this lifesaving discovery was very nearly denied to mankind. And I'm sorry to say the reason is that somebody sat on the research. The trail of evidence clearly shows...

For 7 long years, a billion-dollar drug company covered it up!

What's more, this is undoubtedly not the first time that something like this has happened. Following is a textbook example of how modern drug research works, and how your health falls victim to the pursuit of money and power:

It all started in the early 1990s, when this well-known drug giant started pouring money into the search for a cancer cure...

What gave Jacqueline the power to CONQUER BREAST CANCER?

JACQUELINE HAD BREAST CANCER, but she also had a huge advantage in her battle. Best of all, it works by using your own body's army of natural "killer cells." So, it actually makes you feel more energetic, rather than sapping your strength. Like many such firms, they were intrigued by the healing powers of rainforest plants. They discovered that Graviola was being used by Amazon Indians to treat a huge range of diseases. And when they tested its cancer-fighting powers, bingo, they discovered a revolution...

But you can't make megabucks from any cure UNLESS YOU PATENT IT...

More clinical trials are needed, but more than 20 studies to date have already established that...Graviola can wipe out 12 types of cancer cells, including breast, prostate, colon, lung and pancreatic tumors

Yet, unlike any chemotherapy drug, it leaves healthy cells undamaged.

A miracle? Perhaps. Yet even now, not one drug company we know of has picked it up and run with it.

WHY? Same reason. No one can legally patent it.

Are you starting to see?

AMAZON MIRACLE TREE fights much more than cancer

While scientific research on Graviola has focused on its cancer-fighting powers, the tree has been used for centuries by tribal healers to treat an astonishing array of diseases:

- hypertension
- flu
- ringworm
- rheumatism
- muscle spasm
- diarrhea neuralgia
- scurvy
- malaria
- insomnia
- rashes
- dysentery
- arthritis

The Powers of Graviola (Guanabana in Brazil - Soursop USA)

1) Beats 12 kind of types of cancer such as Breast Cancer, Abdominal Cancer, Ovary Cancer, Uterus Cancer, Lung Cancer, Prostate Cancer, Boon Cancer, Pancreas Cancer, Skin Cancer, Blood Cancer (Leukemia), Bladder Cancer, Liver Cancer

Salubrious way back to a healthy state

2) The Fruit contains a substance called ACETOGENIN that has been proven as 10.000 (ten thousand times) stronger as ACETOGENIN, the drug used for Chemo therapy all over the world with the result of 90% to 10% survivors only - a Bingo Game with the life of people in all nations because the cure is already known.

3) As it is a NUTRIENT it works from INSIDE OUT - eating up the cancer cells, any kind of viruses, bacteria etc. Nutrients have no side effects on our body!!! - unbelievable, miraculous, BUT TRUE (I had the honor to experience many people with cancer even in a very advanced state who were getting well with a Power Juice containing Graviola and there are 1000s in Latin America who had the chance to know about it since 9 years of applications. Solution, Real Cure and permanently heal without Chemo. In case that the doctors ordain Chemo this Special prepared Juice has the powers to protect the healthy cells from burning and allows just the cancer cells to be destroyed, no nausea, no hair loss, neither any other common side effects taking that power plant of healing simultaneously.

GRAVIOLA BENEFITS

The new buzzword in medical therapeutics this wonder plant continues to gain popularity in the developed and developing economies alike. The Brazilian Paw Paw, as it is better connoted is known by various names in different geographies, the more popular ones being Soursop and Sirsak. Soursop is not a recent discovery considering the fact that the plant has been known to mankind for centuries. The Spanish call it Guanabana while the Portuguese call it Graviola. If history is any index, it has been consumed by people the world over to treat a range of disease conditions. Literature indicates that while the Brazilian Amazon women drunk the juice to increase lactation, others used the juice mixed with olive oil as a local application to treat Rheumatism. Thus it is scarcely surprising that Graviola benefits are here to stay.

Concurrently natives of West Indies have used the fruits as well as the juice to treat diarrhoea and fever. The bark and the leaves of the tree are a significant contributor considering that they have proved to be beneficial in the treatment of heart disease, stomach pain and insomnia.

Those with a penchant for facts would find it fascinating that native tribes in the rain forests scatter the crushed seeds around the bed and the pillow so as to ensure a sound sleep at night. If seeking a cure for depression and mental apathy, daily consumption of tea prepared from the leaves of Paw Paw have returned encouraging results like a significant elevation of mood. Thus it is scarcely surprising that this plant has been grown in Central and Southern America for many centuries.

Essentially a small evergreen tree found predominantly in Latin America, the biological name is Anona Muricata Linn and is best classified as a rainforest plant. The root, bark, stems and the fruits are used to make medicines.

Scientists are of the opinion that the bioactive chemicals present in the fruit can selectively kill cancer cells while sparing the healthy variants. Although considered as an effective option for those diagnosed with tumours or cancer, it will take many years for clinical trials to conclude and substantiate such therapeutic benefits. One of the silent killers, hypertension or high blood pressure is best treated by consuming a medicinal tea made from the root, bark and even the leaves.

Although the benefits are many, the plant is not always safe. The cardinal rule being that it is best avoided during pregnancy and lactation as it can damage the brain cells and may even cause disorders of movement. Studies conducted in a Caribbean laboratory have confirmed the presence of a specific chemical called annonacin which can trigger off an attack of atypical Parkinson's.

Finally considering the phenomenal growth in the number of diabetics in the developed economies in recent times, blood sugar control is a major cause for concern. One of the most popular Graviola benefits is the effective control of high blood sugar levels when extracts from the bark and leaves of this plant are ingested.

OTHER KNOWN GRAVIOLA BENEFITS

Aside from what we've mentioned above, other soursop benefits include:

1. Stronger immune system

Soursop has a lot of excellent properties that are necessary to keep your immune system strong. These properties kill free radicals and ensure your immune system is at optimum health so it can effectively perform its functions such as warding off diseases.

2. Regular bowel movements

Graviola is rich in fiber which means that when you consume it regularly, you can expect regular bowel movements. With graviola, you don't have to worry about constipation and hemorrhoids.

3. Increased energy

Soursop has properties that keep your body active and energized so you won't feel lethargic all day.

4. Osteoporosis prevention

Soursop is rich in calcium and phosphorous to help strengthen the bones and prevent bone and joint diseases such as osteoporosis.

5. Heart disease and nerve disease prevention

Because soursop can aid in proper blood circulation, boost metabolism and prevent damage to your nerves, you will have a better functioning heart and your nervous system will also be less likely to get damaged as you grow older.

Although there has not been enough scientific evidence to back up some claims, it's been widely believed that sour sop leaves can also treat gout by lowering the uric acid in the body. Simply boil 6 – 10 leaves with 2 cups of water and drink one cup twice a day. For those suffering from back pain and rheumatism, you can benefit from the use of graviola extract obtained from its leaves, by drinking it hot once a day. Soursop is also believed to help prevent infection by inhibiting the growth of viruses, bacteria and parasites.

What Makes Graviola So Beneficial to the Body?

To understand why there are dozens of graviola benefits, you have to know the composition of this plant. First of all, the soursop fruit is rich in vitamins and minerals including vitamin B1, B2, and C. It also has potassium, calcium, zinc, phosphorous and magnesium. The stem, bark and leaves are rich in antioxidants particularly Coenzyme Q10 to fight inflammation, eliminate free radicals, and ensure your body is functioning at optimum levels.

When you take a look at all the good things present in graviola, it's easy to see why people are eating the fruit, boiling the leaves and even taking graviola capsules. In many ways, the plant makes people healthy and improve their □uality of life.

GRAVIOLA SIDE EFFECTS

But like most remedies and treatments, there are also some side effects to using graviola. Medical experts warn pregnant and lactating women against the use of graviola pills, graviola capsules and fruit. The safety of this supplement to babies and fetus has not been determined.

In addition, there are reports that consuming soursop regularly may put a person at risk of developing Parkinson's disease. However, keep in mind that these findings were obtained using cultured neurons and not human test subjects so the data is not completely accurate.

CONTRAINDICATIONS:

• Graviola has demonstrated uterine stimulant activity in an animal study (rats) and should therefore not be used during pregnancy.

• Graviola has demonstrated hypotensive, vasodilator, and cardiodepressant activities in animal studies and is contraindicated for people with low blood pressure. People taking antihypertensive drugs should check with their doctors before taking graviola and monitor their blood pressure accordingly (as medications may need adjusting).

• Graviola has demonstrated significant in vitro antimicrobial properties. Chronic, long-term use of this plant may lead to die-off of friendly bacteria in the digestive tract due to its antimicrobial properties. Supplementing the diet with probiotics and digestive enzymes is advisable if this plant is used for longer than 30 days.

• Graviola has demonstrated emetic properties in one animal study with pigs. Large single dosages may cause nausea or vomiting. Reduce the usage accordingly if this occurs.

• One study with rats given a stem-bark extract intragastrically (at 100 mg/kg) reported an increase in dopamine, norepinephrine, and monomine oxidase activity, as well as a inhibition of serotonin release in stress-induced rats.

• Alcohol extracts of graviola leaf showed no toxicity or side effects in mice at 100 mg/kg; however, at a dosage of 300 mg/kg, a reduction in explorative behavior and mild abdominal constrictions was observed. If sedation or sleepiness occurs, reduce the amount used.

Other Practitioner Observations:

- Graviola has demonstrated in vitro antimicrobial properties. Chronic, long-term use of this plant might lead to some die-off of friendly bacteria in the digestive tract. Supplementing the diet with probiotics and digestive enzymes may be helpful to counteract this possible effect.

- Graviola has demonstrated emetic properties in one animal study with pigs. Large single dosages may cause nausea or vomiting. Reduce the usage accordingly or take with a meal if nausea occurs.

- Drinking plenty of water (at least 8 glasses a day) is helpful to reduce Herxheimer reactions and flush dead and dying cells from the body.

- One of three documented mechanisms of action of graviola is by decreasing energy to abnormal cells (called an ATP-inhibitor). Taking supplements that increase cellular energy (like CoQ10) will counteract or disable this one mechanism of action of graviola (however, the other two mechanisms of action will be unaffected).

Drug Interactions:

None have been reported; however, graviola may potentiate antihypertensive and cardiac depressant drugs. It may potentiate antidepressant drugs and interfere with MAO-inhibitor drugs.

CONCLUSION

Healing of cancer is possible: knowing about the cause of self creation and with the help of Mother Earth Cancer has no chance!!!!

Within three weeks we had a intestine carcinoma disappearing, one prostate cancer patient who had the surgery marked, he was called into the hospital three days before the marked date for last examinations and o wonder all metastasis had disappeared. The doctors did not belief it and they said that those tumors cannot disappear just like that, that they are certainly hidden in some place and they ordained surgery anyways. Is this normal?

A single mom with an 9 year old girl: after three chemo therapies and surgery -close to death she was in a very advanced state, no hair, no faith, with a lot of fears to let her girl behind alone - after 4 days she started to feel better after 10 days her hair started growing again, after 2 weeks she was sure that she will survive. she said: my doctor will not believe this-at the next examination the result was so amazing that the doctor made a national seminary on her case, but he did not to listen to her how she got better

GRAVIOLA HAS THE POWER TO PREVENT and it is just a fruit in the Garden of Life - reproduced in plantations to let the Rainforest intact......

Made in the
USA
Middletown, DE